THE HEALTHY RECIPES DIET

GOUT

COOKBOOK BIBLE

By Sherrill Freer Smith

The material offered here is claimed to be accurate and comprehensive, and the recipient reader is totally and exclusively responsible for any liability resulting from use or misuse of any policies, processes, or instructions supplied here.

The publisher is not, under any circumstances, legally responsible or liable for any repairs, damages, or financial losses resulting directly or indirectly from the information included herein. The relevant author is the owner of all copies not owned by the publisher.

This page contains unique material that is exclusively provided for educational purposes. Information is presented for free and without any type of guarantee. The trademarks that are utilized do not get any payment, and they are published without the owner's knowledge or permission. All trade names and trademarks mentioned in the book are the sole property of their respective owners and are only used for illustration. The document does not belong to the own

The document is focused on giving precise and reliable information on the topic and issue covered. The general public is advised that the publication is exempt from obligations to provide officially recognized or other qualifying services. A seasoned practitioner in the industry needs to be contacted if legal or professional guidance is required. From a declaration of principles that was accepted and approved by a committee of the American Bar Association and a committee of publishers and associations. Any part of the document, whether it is in printed or electronic form, cannot be copied, duplicated, or transferred. Without the publisher's previous written approval, it is completely forbidden to reproduce the publication, and all changes must be made in writing. Everything has a place.

Table of Contents

Introduction

Welcome to "The New Healthy Recipes Gout Diet Cookbook Bible"! In this comprehensive guide, we bring you a collection of 40 plus delicious and nutritious recipes specifically tailored for individuals who wants to cure gout, along with a convenient 14-day meal plan to help you on your journey to better health. Gout is a form of inflammatory arthritis. It occurs when uric acid crystals accumulate in one (or rarely several) of the body's joints. This painful condition often comes on without warning and most commonly affects the base of the big toe.

Gout can cause severe pain, inflammation, and difficulty walking if left untreated.

This book will detail the causes, diagnosis, and treatment strategies for this arthritic condition.

Gout can be treated and managed with medications and healthy lifestyle habits. Your doctor or nutritionist can help you develop the best treatment strategy for you. The heart of this cookbook lies in its diverse and flavorful recipes. We have meticulously curated a collection that encompasses a wide range of culinary traditions, ensuring that there is something for everyone. From refreshing salads and hearty soups to mouthwatering main dishes and delectable desserts, you will discover new favorites that align with your gout diet.

To help you plan your meals and stay on track, we have included a 14-day meal plan that takes the guesswork out of your dietary choices. Each day is carefully balanced, incorporating a variety of ingredients and flavors, while ensuring that you stay within the guidelines of a gout-friendly diet.

"The New Healthy Recipes Gout Diet Cookbook Bible" is not just a cookbook; it is a guide to transforming your relationship with food. By adopting these recipes and the principles behind them, you can take charge of your health and manage your gout effectively.

We invite you to embark on this culinary journey with us, embracing a new way of eating that nourishes both your body and your taste buds. Get ready to savor the flavors, explore new ingredients, and experience the joy of cooking meals that promote well-being. Let this cookbook be your trusted companion as you embark on a path to a healthier, more fulfilling life.

Remember, managing gout doesn't mean sacrificing taste. With "The New Healthy Recipes Gout Diet Cookbook Bible," you can indulge in delicious meals while taking care of your health. Get ready to embark on a flavorful adventure that will transform the way you eat and live. Living with gout can be challenging, as the condition demands careful attention to what we eat and drink. Gout is a form of arthritis caused by the accumulation of uric acid crystals in the joints, leading to inflammation, pain, and discomfort. While medication plays a crucial role in managing gout, adopting a gout-friendly diet is equally vital for maintaining a healthy lifestyle.

"The New Healthy Recipes Gout Diet Cookbook Bible" is here to simplify your gout-friendly culinary experience without compromising on taste or variety. We believe that eating healthy should never be boring or restrictive. That's why our team of expert chefs and nutritionists has meticulously curated a collection of recipes that are not only suitable for gout sufferers but also bursting with flavors and textures that will tantalize your taste buds.

Within the pages of this cookbook, you will discover a wide range of recipes, including appetizers, main courses, side dishes, snacks, and even indulgent desserts – all tailored to support a gout-friendly diet. Each recipe has been carefully crafted with a focus on ingredients known to be beneficial for managing gout, such as low-purine foods, anti-inflammatory ingredients, and an abundance of fresh fruits and vegetables.

Overeiw of Gout

In conclusion, "The New Healthy Recipes Gout Diet Cookbook Bible" offers a comprehensive and practical approach to managing gout through delicious and nutritious meals. With a collection of 100 recipes and a well-structured 14-day meal plan, this cookbook serves as a valuable resource for individuals looking to improve their health and minimize gout-related symptoms.

By focusing on ingredients that are known to alleviate gout and promoting a balanced diet, this book empowers readers to take control of their condition and make positive dietary choices. Each recipe is carefully crafted to not only satisfy taste buds but also provide essential nutrients and reduce purine intake.

The 14-day meal plan simplifies the process of transitioning to a gout-friendly diet, offering a clear roadmap for success. Whether you're a beginner or an experienced cook, the cookbook provides step-by-step instructions and helpful tips to ensure that each dish is prepared with ease and confidence.

"The New Healthy Recipes Gout Diet Cookbook Bible" goes beyond mere recipes; it serves as a guide to understanding the principles behind a gout-friendly diet and the impact of food choices on overall health. With this knowledge in hand, readers can make informed decisions about their meals and develop sustainable habits for long-term well-being.

In summary, this cookbook is a valuable companion for anyone seeking to improve their health and manage gout effectively. By combining delicious recipes, a well-designed meal plan, and insightful information, it equips individuals with the tools they need to lead a healthier and happier life.

Gout is a general term for a variety of conditions caused by a buildup of uric acid. This buildup usually affects the feet.

If you have gout, you'll probably feel swelling and pain in the joints of your foot, particularly your big toe. Sudden and intense pain, or gout attacks, can make it feel like your foot is on fire.

Symptoms of gout

Some people have too much uric acid in their blood but no symptoms. This is called asymptomatic hyperuricemia.

For acute gout, symptoms come on quickly from the buildup of uric acid crystals in your joint and last for 3 to 10 days.
You'll have intense pain and swelling, and your joint may feel warm. Between gout attacks, you won't have any symptoms.

If you don't treat gout, it can become chronic. Hard lumps called tophi can eventually develop in your joints and the skin and soft tissue surrounding them. These deposits can permanently damage your joints.

Prompt treatment is important to prevent gout from turning chronic.

Gout home remedies

Some home remedies may help lower uric acid levels and prevent gout attacks. The following foods and drinks have been suggested for gout:

- tart cherries
- magnesium
- ginger
- diluted apple cider vinegar
- celery
- nettle tea
- dandelion
- milk thistle seeds

But these alone may not be enough to manage gout.

If left untreated, gout can eventually lead to gouty arthritis, which is a more severe form of arthritis. This painful condition can leave your joint permanently damaged and swollen.

The treatment plan your doctor recommends will depend on the stage and severity of your gout.

Medications to treat gout work in one of two ways: They relieve pain and bring down inflammation, or they prevent future gout attacks by lowering uric acid levels.

Drugs to relieve gout pain include:

- nonsteroidal anti-inflammatory drugs (NSAIDs), such as aspirin (Bufferin), ibuprofen (Advil, Motrin), and naproxen (Aleve)
- colchicine (Colcrys, Mitigare)
- corticosteroids

Drugs that prevent gout attacks include:

- xanthine oxidase inhibitors, such as allopurinol (Lopurin, Zyloprim) and febuxostat (Uloric)
- probenecid (Probalan)

Along with medications, your doctor may recommend lifestyle changes to help manage your symptoms and reduce your risk of future gout attacks. For example, your doctor may encourage you to:

- reduce your alcohol intake, if you drink
- lose weight, if you're overweight

- quit smoking, if you smoke

In addition a few complementary therapies have also shown promise.

Gout surgery

Gout can typically be treated without surgery. But after many years, this condition can damage the joints, tear the tendons, and cause infections in the skin over the joints.

Hard deposits, called tophi, can build up on your joints and in other places, like your ear. These lumps may be painful and swollen, and they can permanently damage your joints.

Three surgical procedures treat tophi:

- tophi removal surgery

- joint fusion surgery

- joint replacement surgery

Which one of these surgeries your doctor recommends depends on the extent of the damage, where the tophi are located, and your personal preferences.

Causes of gout

The buildup of uric acid in your blood from the breakdown of purines causes gout.
Certain conditions, such as blood and metabolism disorders or dehydration, make your body produce too much uric acid.

A kidney or thyroid problem, or an inherited disorder, can make it harder for your body to remove excess uric acid.

You're more likely to get gout if you:

- are a middle-aged man or postmenopausal woman
- have parents, siblings, or other family members with gout
- drink alcohol
- take medications such as diuretics and cyclosporine
- have a condition like high blood pressure, kidney disease, thyroid disease, diabetes, or sleep apnea

For some people, gout is caused by consuming foods that are high in gout-producing purines.

Foods to avoid

Certain foods are naturally high in purines, which your body breaks down into uric acid.

Most people can tolerate high-purine foods. But if your body has trouble releasing excess uric acid, you may want to avoid certain foods and drinks, such as:

- red meats
- organ meats
- certain seafood
- alcohol
- Sugar-sweetened beverages and foods containing the sugar fructose can also be problematic, even though they don't contain purines.

Some foods help reduce uric acid levels in the body and are good choices if you have gout.

Gout and alcohol

Alcohol, like red meat and seafood, is high in purines. When your body breaks down purines, the process releases uric acid.

More uric acid increases your risk of having gout. Alcohol can also reduce the rate at which your body removes uric acid.

Not everyone who drinks will develop gout. But a high consumption of alcohol (more than 12 drinks per week) can increase the risk — especially in men. Beer is more likely than liquor to influence the risk.

In surveys, people have reported that drinking alcohol triggers their gout flare-ups.

Gout diagnosis

Your doctor can diagnose gout based on a review of your medical history, a physical exam, and your symptoms. Your doctor will likely base your diagnosis on:

- your description of your joint pain
- how often you've experienced intense pain in your joint
- how red or swollen the area is

Your doctor may also order a test to check for a buildup of uric acid in your joint. A sample of fluid taken from your joint can show whether it contains uric acid. They may also want to take an X-ray of your joint.

If you have symptoms of gout, you can start with a visit to your primary care doctor. If your gout is severe, you may need to see a specialist in joint diseases.

If you need help finding a primary care doctor, then check out our FindCare tool here.

Gout triggers

Certain foods, medications, and conditions can set off gout symptoms. You may need to avoid or limit foods and drinks like these, which are high in purines:

- red meat, such as pork and veal
- organ meats
- fish, such as cod, scallops, mussels, and salmon
- alcohol

- sodas

- fruit juice

Some medications you take to manage other conditions increase the level of uric acid in your blood. Talk with your doctor if you take any of these drugs:

- diuretics, or water pills

- aspirin

- blood pressure-lowering medications, such as beta-blockers and angiotensin II receptor blockers

Your health may also be a factor in flare-ups. All of these conditions have been linked to gout:

- obesity

- diabetes or prediabetes

- dehydration

- joint injury

- infections

- congestive heart failure

- high blood pressure

- kidney disease

Sometimes it can be hard to pinpoint which of these factors is behind your gout attacks. Keeping a diary is one way to track your diet, medications, and health to help identify the cause of your symptoms.

Gout prevention

Here are a few steps you can take to help prevent gout:

- Limit how much alcohol you drink.

- Limit how much purine-rich food, such as shellfish, lamb, beef, pork, and organ meat, you eat.

- Eat a low-fat, nondairy diet that's rich in vegetables.

- Maintain a healthy weight.

- Avoid smoking.

- Exercise regularly.

- Stay hydrated.

If you have medical conditions or take medications that raise your risk of gout, ask your doctor how you can lower your risk of gout attacks.

Gout with tophus

When uric acid crystals build up in joints for a long time, they produce hard deposits called tophi under the skin. Without treatment, these tophi can damage bone and cartilage and leave the joints permanently disfigured.

Tophi are swollen lumps around the joints that look like knots on a tree trunk. They occur in joints like the fingers, feet, and knees, as well as on the ears. Tophi themselves don't hurt, but the inflammation they cause can be painful.

Sometimes tophi form in connective tissue outside the joints.

Is gout painful?

Yes, gout can be painful. In fact, pain in the big toe is often one of the first symptoms people report. The pain is accompanied by more typical arthritis symptoms, such as swelling and warmth in the joints.

Gout pain can vary in severity. Pain in the big toe can be very intense at first. After the acute attack, it may subside to a dull ache.

The pain, as well as swelling and other symptoms, are the result of the body launching a defense (by the immune system) against uric acid crystals in the joints. This attack leads to the release of chemicals called cytokines, which promote painful inflammation.

Gout essential oils

Essential oils are plant-based substances used in aromatherapy. Some oils are thought to have anti-inflammatory, pain-relieving, and antibacterial effects.

Some of the essential oils used to treat gout include:

- lemongrass oil

- celery seed oil

- yarrow oil extract

- olive leaf extract

- Chinese cinnamon

Talk with your doctor before you begin using any essential oil. Be aware that the Food and Drug Administration (FDA) doesn't regulate the purity or quality of essential oils, so research the brand.

Be sure to follow these safety precautions when using essential oils:

- Don't put essential oils directly on your skin. It's important to dilute them first with a carrier oil such as coconut oil or jojoba oil. For example, for a 3 percent dilution, mix 20 drops of the essential oil with 6 teaspoons of the carrier oil.

- Don't put essential oils in your mouth, since they're not safe to ingest.

- Store essential oils and carrier oils in a cool, dark place, away from sunlight and heat.

Is gout hereditary?

Gout is at least partly due to heredity. Researchers have found dozens of genes that increase people's susceptibility to gout, including SLC2A9 and ABCG2. Genes associated with gout affect the amount of uric acid the body holds onto and releases.

Because of genetic factors, gout runs in families. People with a parent, sibling, or other close relative who has gout are more likely to get this condition themselves.

It's likely that genes only set the stage for gout. Environmental factors, such as diet, actually trigger the disease.

Gout is a painful arthritic condition that's caused by a buildup of uric acid a waste product in your blood.

Usually, uric acid is removed through your urine when you pee. But when uric acid builds up, it can form sharp crystalsTrusted Source that cause swelling and inflammation in your joints, especially the feet.

Here are common symptoms to look out for along with where and when they typically appear.

Common symptoms of gout

Pain and swelling are the main symptomsTrusted Source of gout, but how these symptoms appear can be rather specific. Gout usually appears as flare-ups with:

- intense or sharp pain

- swelling

- redness

- skin that is hot to the touch

In many cases, gout begins at nightTrusted Source and is so severe that it wakes you from your sleep.

Severe cases may also include bulging or deformed joints. Your doctor will be able to see evidence of uric acid crystalsTrusted Source in the affected joint using an X-ray, ultrasound, or dual-energy CT when making a diagnosis. Taking fluid from the joint and observing uric acid crystals in immune cells may be needed to confirm a gout diagnosis.

Gout is a chronic condition, but it's not always consistent. Flare-ups can last for days to weeks, but you can also have weeks or even years without a flare-up.

Usually, flare-ups targetTrusted Source a single joint, and the big toe is a favored spot for uric acid to collect. Other common places for gout pain include:

- other toe joints
- ankles
- knees

Gout triggers and risk factors

Gout symptoms and flare-ups can be managed. First, it's important to identify triggers and risk factors like:

- obesity

- being assigned male at birth

- heart failure

- high blood pressure

- diabetes

- kidney disease

- diuretic medications

- alcohol

- sugary foods and drinks

- purine-rich foods like red meat, organ meats, and some seafoods

Once you've identified what triggers your gout and any risk factors that you have, you can work with your doctor to create a plan that helps you avoid triggers and manage any medical conditions that affect your condition.

Stay hydrated: Drink plenty of water to help flush out uric acid and prevent the formation of gout crystals.

Follow a gout-friendly diet: Limit your intake of purine-rich foods like organ meats, seafood, and alcohol. Focus on a diet rich in fruits, vegetables, whole grains, and low-fat dairy products.

Apply ice packs: Apply ice packs to the affected joint to reduce inflammation and provide pain relief.

Elevate the affected joint: Elevate the affected joint to help reduce swelling and promote circulation.

Use cherries or cherry juice: Cherries and cherry juice have been shown to help reduce gout attacks. Consume them regularly to help manage symptoms.

Take over-the-counter pain relievers: Nonsteroidal anti-inflammatory drugs (NSAIDs), such as ibuprofen, can help relieve pain and reduce inflammation. However, consult with a healthcare professional before taking any medication.

Maintain a healthy weight: Excess weight can contribute to gout symptoms. Aim for a healthy weight through regular exercise and a balanced diet.

Limit alcohol consumption: Alcohol can increase uric acid levels in the body, leading to gout flare-ups. Minimize or avoid alcohol intake, especially beer and spirits.

Apply a warm compress: After the initial inflammation has subsided, applying a warm compress can help ease joint stiffness and discomfort.

Follow a balanced diet: Opt for a low-purine diet that includes foods like cherries, berries, leafy greens

Use over-the-counter pain relievers: Nonsteroidal anti-inflammatory drugs (NSAIDs) like ibuprofen can help reduce pain and inflammation. However, consult your doctor before taking any medication.

Gout traditional treatments

Treatments for gout are designed to reduce either the pain and inflammation of individual attacks or the frequency of attacks. Traditional treatments include making dietary changes and taking certain medications.

Diet modification

Adjusting your diet is one of the most important ways to reduce the number of acute gout attacks you experience. The goal of these changes is to lower blood levels of uric acid.

The following dietary changes can reduce gout symptoms:

- Reduce or eliminate alcohol, especially beer.

- Drink lots of water or other nonalcoholic beverages.

- Eat more low-fat or nonfat dairy products.

- Avoid high-purine foods, including organ meats (kidneys, liver, and sweetbreads) and oily fish (sardines, anchovies, and herring).

- Limit meat in favor of plant-based proteins like beans and legumes.

- Eat complex carbohydrates, such as whole-grain breads, fruits, and vegetables, rather than sugary sweets and refined carbohydrates like white bread.

Medications

Here's a brief rundown of several classes of drugs used to treat gout:

- Nonsteroidal anti-inflammatory drugs (NSAIDs), corticosteroids, and colchicine all reduce the pain and inflammation associated with an acute gout attack.
- Xanthine oxidase inhibitors like allopurinol reduce the amount of uric acid produced by the body.
- Probenecid improves the kidneys' ability to remove uric acid from the blood.

Gout drugs

During an acute gout attack, the main priority of drug treatment is to reduce pain and inflammation. There are three categories of drugs used for this: NSAIDs, colchicine, and corticosteroids. Two other types of medications are taken daily to help prevent future gout attacks: xanthine oxidase inhibitors and probenecid.

NSAIDs

Nonsteroidal anti-inflammatory drugs (NSAIDs) reduce both pain and inflammation. Many NSAIDs are available over the counter at low doses and at higher doses by prescription. They can cause gastrointestinal side effects, such as nausea, diarrhea, and stomach ulcers. In rare cases, they can cause kidney or liver damage.

NSAIDs commonly used for gout include:

- aspirin (Bufferin)
- celecoxib (Celebrex)
- ibuprofen (Advil)
- indomethacin (Indocin)
- ketoprofen
- naproxen (Aleve)

Colchicine

Colchicine (Colcrys) is a drug used mainly to treat gout. It prevents uric acid in the body from forming urate crystals. If taken very soon after the onset of acute gout symptoms, it can effectively prevent pain and swelling. It's also sometimes prescribed for daily use to prevent future attacks.

However, colchicine also causes side effects including nausea, vomiting, and diarrhea. It's usually prescribed to people who can't take NSAIDs.

Corticosteroids

Corticosteroids are very effective at reducing inflammation. They can be taken orally or injected directly into the affected joint on intravenously. They have serious side effects when used for long periods, including:

- diabetes
- osteoporosis
- high blood pressure
- cataracts
- increased risk of infection
- death of bone tissue (avascular necrosis) especially in the hip and shoulder joints

For this reason, they're generally used only by people who can't take NSAIDs or colchicine. Corticosteroids used for gout include:

- dexamethasone (DexPak)
- methylprednisolone (Medrol)
- prednisolone (Omnipred)
- prednisone (Rayos)

- triamcinolone (Aristospan)

Xanthine oxidase inhibitors

Xanthine oxidase inhibitors reduce the amount of uric acid produced by the body.

However, these drugs can trigger an acute gout attack when you start taking them. They can also make an acute attack worse if they're taken during the attack. For this reason, people with gout are commonly prescribed a short course of colchicine when starting a xanthine oxidase inhibitor.

Side effects of these drugs include rash and nausea.

There are two main xanthine oxidase inhibitors used for gout:

- allopurinol (Lopurin, Zyloprim)

- febuxostat (Uloric)

Probenecid

Probenecid (Probalan) is a drug that helps the kidneys remove uric acid from the blood more effectively. Side effects include rash, upset stomach, and kidney stones.

Gout alternative treatments

Alternative treatments for gout aim either to reduce pain during attacks or to lower uric acid levels and potentially prevent attacks. As with many alternative treatments for any disease or condition, opinions are often mixed as to how well such treatment methods work. Research is often minimal in comparison to traditional medical treatments for gout.

However, many people have had success in using alternative treatments in the management of many diseases and conditions, including gout. Before trying any gout alternative treatments, you should always check with your doctor to be sure that the methods are safe and right for you.

Foods, herbs, and supplements

The following have shown at least some promise for gout.

Coffee. According to the Mayo Clinic, there's evidence that drinking a moderate amount of coffee a day can lower gout risk.

Antioxidant-rich fruits. Dark-colored fruits like blackberries, blueberries, grapes, raspberries, and especially cherries can help keep uric acid under control.

Vitamin C. Consuming moderate amounts of vitamin C is also connected to lower uric acid levels. However, very large doses of the vitamin can actually raise uric acid levels.

Other supplements. There are also herbal supplements that have been found to effectively reduce inflammation including devil's claw, bromelain, and turmeric. These haven't been specifically studied for gout, but they may help with the swelling and pain associated with an attack.

Acupuncture

This technique, which is a form of traditional Chinese medicine, involves placing very thin needles in points on the body. It has been found effective in treating different types of chronic pain. There haven't yet been any studies done on acupuncture and gout, but its pain-relieving properties are promising.

Hot and cold compresses

Switching between a hot compress for three minutes and a cold compress for 30 seconds on the affected area can help reduce pain and swelling that occurs during a gout attack.

Gout prevention

In most people, a first acute gout attack comes without warning, and there aren't any other symptoms of high uric acid. Prevention efforts for gout are focused on preventing future attacks or lessening their severity.

Medication

Xanthine oxidase inhibitors and probenecid both prevent gout attacks by reducing the amount of uric acid in the blood. A doctor may also prescribe an NSAID or colchicine to be taken every day to help make future attacks less painful.

Dietary changes

Careful dietary monitoring can also help to reduce uric acid levels. Your doctor and dietitian can help you create a specific plan, but here are some of the most common changes should make:

- Drink more water and other nonalcoholic fluids.
- Drink less alcohol, especially beer.
- Eat less meat.
- Limit high-purine meats and seafood.
- Limit added sugars and sodas.
- Increase intake of fruits, vegetables, legumes and whole grains.

Some gout is described as gouty arthritis and therefore may benefit from dietary changes similar to those recommended for arthritis sufferers, like avoidance of gluten-containing foods and dairy.

Maintaining a healthy weight

In addition, dietary changes may also have the goal of reducing body weight. Obesity is a risk factor for gout. Maintaining a healthy weight through a balanced diet and regular exercise can help prevent attacks.

Natural Home Remedies for Gout

Plenty of options are available for helping or preventing gout attacks at home. Most are natural and have little to no side effects. But in some cases, you will need to get medical help.

Gout is a type of arthritis that causes pain similar to osteoarthritis, though there are some distinct differences.

It's caused by high uric acid buildup in the blood. Uric acid then accumulates in joints, causing inflammation with discomfort and pain.

Some natural remedies may help. However, if your gout pain is very sudden or intense, contact your doctor before trying any of the remedies below.

Natural remedies for gout

Cherries or tart cherry juice

According to a 2016 surveyTrusted Source, cherries whether sour, sweet, red, black, in extract form, as a juice, or raw are a very popular and potentially successful home remedy for many.

One 2012 study and another that same year also suggest cherries may work to prevent gout attacks.

This research recommends three servings of any cherry form over a two-day period, which was considered the most effective.

Magnesium

Magnesium is a dietary mineral. Some claim it's good for gout because deficiency of magnesium may worsen chronic inflammatory stress in the body, though no studies prove this.

Still, a 2015 studyTrusted Source showed that adequate magnesium is associated with lower and healthier levels of uric acid, thus potentially lowering gout risk. This applied to men but not women within the study.

Try taking magnesium supplements, but read label directions closely. Or, eat magnesium-rich foods daily. This may decrease gout risk or gout occurrence long term.

Ginger

Ginger is a culinary food and herb prescribed for inflammatory conditions. Its ability to help gout is well-documented.

One study found topical ginger reduced pain related to uric acid in gout. Another study showed that in subjects with high levels of uric acid (hyperuricemia), their serum uric acid level was reduced by ginger. But the subjects were rats, and ginger was taken internally rather than topically.

Make a ginger compress or paste by boiling water with 1 tablespoon of grated fresh gingerroot. Soak a washcloth in the mixture. When cool, apply the washcloth to the area where you're experiencing pain at least once per day for 15 to 30 minutes. Skin irritation is possible, so it's best to do a test on a small patch of skin first.

Take ginger internally by boiling water and steeping 2 teaspoons of gingerroot for 10 minutes. Enjoy 3 cups per day.

Interactions are possible. Let your doctor know first before you take large amounts of ginger.

Warm water with apple cider vinegar, lemon juice, and turmeric

Apple cider vinegar, lemon juice, and turmeric are each frequently recommended anecdotally for gout. Together, they make a pleasant beverage and remedy.

No strong research supports apple cider vinegar for gout, though studies show it may support the kidneys. Otherwise, research is promising for lemon juice and turmeric for lowering uric acid.

Mix juice from one squeezed half lemon into warm water. Combine with 2 teaspoons turmeric and 1 teaspoon apple cider vinegar. Adjust to taste. Drink two to three times per day.

Celery or celery seeds

Celery is a food traditionally used to treat urinary issues. For gout, extract and seeds of the vegetable have become popular home remedies.

Experimental use is well-documented, though scientific research is scant. It's thought that celery may reduce inflammation.

Adequate celery amounts for treating gout aren't documented. Try eating celery many times per day, especially raw celery sticks, juice, extract, or seeds.

If purchasing an extract or supplement, follow label directions closely.

Nettle tea

Stinging nettle (Urtica dioica) is an herbal remedy for gout that may reduce inflammation and pain.

Traditional use is frequently referred to in studies. There's still no research directly proving it works. One study showed it protected the kidneys, but the subjects were male rabbits, and kidney injury was induced by administration of gentamicin, an antibiotic.

To try this tea, brew a cup by boiling water. Steep 1 to 2 teaspoons of dried nettle per cup of water. Drink up to 3 cups per day.

Dandelion

Dandelion teas, extracts, and supplements are used to improve liver and kidney health.

They may lower uric acid levels in those at risk for kidney injury, as shown in a 2013 study and a 2016 study, but these were on rats. Dandelion is unproven to help gout.

You can use dandelion tea, an extract, or a supplement. Follow label directions closely.

Milk thistle seeds

Milk thistle is an herb used for liver health.

A 2016 study suggested it may lower uric acid in the midst of conditions that can hurt the kidneys, and another from 2013 supports it. However, both studies were on rats.

Follow dosing directions on a milk thistle supplement carefully or discuss it with your doctor.

Hibiscus

Hibiscus is a garden flower, food, tea, and traditional herbal remedy.

It may be a folk remedy used to treat gout. One study showed that hibiscus might lower uric acid levels, though this study was performed on rats.

Use a supplement, tea, or extract. Follow label directions closely.

Topical cold or hot application

Applying cold or hot water to inflamed joints may also be effective.

Studies and opinions on this are mixed. Soaking in cold water is most often recommended and considered most effective. Ice packs may also work.

Soaking in hot water is typically only recommended when inflammation isn't as intense.

Alternating hot and cold applications may also be helpful.

Apples

Natural health sites may recommend apples as part of gout-reducing diets. The claim: Apples contain malic acid, which lowers uric acid.

However, there aren't any studies supporting this for gout. Apples also contain fructose, which may trigger hyperuricemia, leading to gout flare-ups.

Eating one apple per day is good for overall health. It may be mildly beneficial for gout, but only if it doesn't add to excessive daily sugar consumption.

Bananas

Bananas are thought to be good for gout. They're potassium-rich, which helps the tissue and organs in the body to function properly.

Bananas also contain sugars, including fructose, which can be a gout trigger. Many foods are higher in potassium and lower in sugar than bananas, such as dark leafy greens and avocados.

Eat one banana per day for benefit. No studies yet support any benefit from bananas for gout.

Epsom salts

Some people recommend a bath of Epsom salts to prevent gout attacks.

The idea is that Epsom salts are rich in magnesium, which may lower gout risk. However, studies show magnesium can't be adequately absorbed through skin to confer any health benefits.

To give Epsom salts a try, mix 1 to 2 cups in your bath. Soak your entire body or only specific joints for symptom relief.

Other tips for reducing gout flare-ups

Eliminate diet triggers

Diet is often closely related to gout flareups and pain. Avoiding triggers and keeping to a good gout diet is an important remedy in and of itself.

Studies show red meat, seafood, sugar, and alcohol are the most likely triggers. Stick to low-sugar fruits, vegetables, whole grains, nuts, legumes, and low-fat dairy instead.

Hydrate often

Drinking plenty of water is important to kidney function. Keeping the kidneys in good shape can also reduce uric acid crystal buildup and gout attacks.

Make sure to stay hydrated and drink plenty of water, which can be helpful for gout. No studies show it can replace gout treatments, however.

Get plenty of rest

Gout attacks can interfere with movement and mobility.

To avoid worsening symptoms, relax and stay put while joints are inflamed. Avoid exercising, bearing heavy weights, and using joints excessively, which can worsen the pain and duration of a flare-up.

Recipes for Gout

Breakfast

Oatmeal with Nuts and Berries

Ingredients:

- 1/2 cup rolled oats
- 1 cup water or milk
- 1 tablespoon chopped walnuts
- 1 tablespoon fresh blueberries
- 1 tablespoon fresh raspberries
- 1 teaspoon honey

Instructions:

- Cook oats in water or milk until soft. Top with walnuts, berries, and drizzle with honey.

Greek Yogurt Parfait

Ingredients:

1 cup Greek yogurt

1/4 cup granola

1/4 cup diced mango

1 tablespoon chia seeds

Instructions:

- Layer Greek yogurt, granola, mango, and chia seeds in a glass or bowl. Repeat the layers and serve.

- Egg White and Veggie Omelette

Ingredients:

- 3 egg whites
- 1/4 cup chopped bell peppers
- 1/4 cup chopped spinach
- 1/4 cup diced tomatoes
- Salt and pepper to taste

Instructions:

- Whisk egg whites with salt and pepper. Pour into a heated and greased pan. Add veggies and cook until set.

Chia Seed Pudding

Ingredients:

- 2 tablespoons chia seeds
- 1 cup unsweetened almond milk
- 1/2 teaspoon vanilla extract
- 1 tablespoon chopped almonds
- Fresh strawberries, for garnish

Instructions:

- Mix chia seeds, almond milk, and vanilla extract. Refrigerate for at least 4 hours or overnight. Top with chopped almonds and strawberries before serving.

Fruit Salad with Mint

Ingredients:

- 1 cup diced watermelon
- 1 cup diced pineapple
- 1 cup diced cantaloupe
- Fresh mint leaves, chopped

Instructions:

- Toss all the fruits together in a bowl. Garnish with chopped mint leaves.

Sweet Potato Hash

Ingredients:

- 1 medium sweet potato, grated
- 1/4 cup diced onion
- 1/4 cup diced bell peppers
- 1 tablespoon olive oil
- Salt and pepper to taste

Instructions:

- Heat olive oil in a skillet. Add sweet potato, onion, and bell peppers. Cook until tender, season with salt and pepper.

Cottage Cheese and Berries

Ingredients:

- 1/2 cup low-fat cottage cheese
- 1/4 cup fresh strawberries
- 1/4 cup fresh blueberries
- 1 tablespoon honey

Instructions:

- Top cottage cheese with strawberries, blueberries, and drizzle with honey.

Banana Nut Muffins

Ingredients:

- 1 cup mashed ripe bananas
- 1/4 cup honey
- 1/4 cup unsweetened applesauce
- 1 egg
- 1 1/2 cups whole wheat flour
- 1/4 cup chopped walnuts
- 1 teaspoon baking powder
- 1/2 teaspoon baking soda
- 1/2 teaspoon cinnamon

Instructions:

- Preheat oven to 350°F (175°C). Mix all the ingredients in a bowl. Pour into muffin cups and bake for 20-25 minutes.

- Spinach and Feta Egg Muffins
- Ingredients:
- 6 eggs
- 1/4 cup diced spinach
- 1/4 cup crumbled feta cheese
- Salt and pepper to taste

Instructions:

- Preheat oven to 350°F (175°C). Whisk eggs with salt and pepper. Stir in spinach and feta. Pour into greased muffin cups and bake for 15-18 minutes.

Vegetable Frittata:

Ingredients:

- 4 eggs
- 1 cup mixed vegetables (bell peppers, zucchini, onions, etc.), diced
- ¼ cup shredded low-fat cheese
- Salt and pepper to taste
- 1 teaspoon olive oil

Instructions:

- Preheat the oven to 350°F (175°C).
- Heat olive oil in an oven-safe skillet over medium heat.
- Add the diced vegetables and sauté until slightly tender.

- In a bowl, whisk the eggs and season with salt and pepper.
- Pour the egg mixture over the vegetables in the skillet.
- Sprinkle shredded cheese on top.
- Transfer the skillet to the preheated oven and bake for about 15-20 minutes, or until the frittata is set.
- Slice into wedges and serve.

Overnight Oats:

Ingredients:

- ½ cup rolled oats
- ½ cup unsweetened almond milk
- 1 tablespoon chia seeds
- 1 tablespoon honey or maple syrup
- Fresh berries or sliced banana for topping

Instructions:

- In a jar or bowl, combine rolled oats, almond milk, chia seeds, and honey/maple syrup.
- Stir well, cover, and refrigerate overnight.
- In the morning, give it a good stir, and top with fresh berries or sliced banana.

Smoked Salmon Wrap:

Ingredients:

- 1 whole wheat tortilla or wrap
- 2 ounces smoked salmon
- 2 tablespoons low-fat cream cheese

- Thinly sliced cucumber
- Fresh dill (opt)

Instructions:

- Spread cream cheese on the tortilla or wrap.
- Place smoked salmon, cucumber slices, and fresh dill on top.
- Roll up the wrap tightly and slice in half.
- Serve and enjoy.

Greek Yogurt Parfait:

Ingredients:

- ½ cup low-fat Greek yogurt
- ¼ cup granola (low sugar)
- ¼ cup fresh berries
- 1 tablespoon chopped almonds or walnuts
- 1 teaspoon honey

Instructions:

- In a glass or bowl, layer Greek yogurt, granola, fresh berries, and chopped nuts.
- Drizzle honey over the top.
- Repeat the layers if desired.
- Enjoy your parfait.

Vegetable Oatmeal:

Ingredients:

- ½ cup rolled oats
- 1 cup vegetable broth
- ¼ cup diced mixed vegetables (carrots, peas, bell peppers, etc.)
- Salt and pepper to taste
- Fresh parsley for garnish

Instructions:

- In a saucepan, bring the vegetable broth to a boil.
- Add the rolled oats and diced vegetables.
- Reduce heat and simmer until the oats are cooked and the vegetables are tender.
- Season with salt and pepper.
- Transfer to a bowl and garnish with fresh parsley.

Berry Smoothie:

Ingredients:

- 1 cup unsweetened almond milk
- 1 cup fresh or frozen mixed berries
- ½ banana
- 1 tablespoon almond butter
- 1 teaspoon honey (optional)
- Ice cubes (if using fresh berries)

Instructions:

- Place all the ingredients in a blender.
- Blend until smooth and creamy.
- Taste and add honey if desired.
- Pour into a glass and serve chilled.

Egg and Veggie Muffins:

Ingredients:

- 4 eggs
- ½ cup diced mixed vegetables (spinach, tomatoes, onions, etc.)
- ¼ cup shredded low-fat cheese
- Salt and pepper to taste
- Cooking spray

Instructions:

- Preheat the oven to 350°F (175°C) and grease a muffin tin with cooking spray.
- In a bowl, whisk the eggs and season with salt and pepper.
- Stir in the diced vegetables and shredded cheese.
- Pour the mixture into the greased muffin tin, filling each cup about ¾ full.
- Bake for 15-20 minutes or until the muffins are set and golden.
- Remove from the oven, let cool slightly, and remove from the tin.
- Serve warm or refrigerate for later.

Cottage Cheese Pancakes:

Ingredients:

- ½ cup cottage cheese
- 2 eggs
- ¼ cup whole wheat flour
- 1 tablespoon honey or maple syrup
- ½ teaspoon vanilla extract
- Cooking spray

Instructions:

- In a blender or food processor, combine cottage cheese, eggs, whole wheat flour, honey/maple syrup, and vanilla extract.
- Blend until smooth.
- Heat a non-stick skillet over medium heat and coat with cooking spray.
- Pour about ¼ cup of the batter onto the skillet to form each pancake.
- Cook for 2-3 minutes on each side until golden brown.
- Repeat with the remaining batter.
- Serve with your choice of fruit or a dollop of Greek yogurt.

Turkey Sausage Breakfast Burrito:

Ingredients:

- 1 whole wheat tortilla or wrap
- 2 turkey sausage links, cooked and sliced
- 2 eggs, scrambled

- ¼ cup diced bell peppers
- 2 tablespoons shredded low-fat cheese
- Salt and pepper to taste

Instructions:

- Heat a non-stick skillet over medium heat.
- Cook the scrambled eggs and diced bell peppers together until the eggs are cooked through.
- Place the tortilla or wrap on a plate and layer the cooked eggs, sliced turkey sausage, and shredded cheese in the center.
- Season with salt and pepper.
- Roll up the tortilla tightly, folding in the sides.
- Slice in half and enjoy.

Green Smoothie Bowl:

Ingredients:

- 1 frozen banana
- 1 cup fresh spinach
- ½ cup unsweetened almond milk
- 1 tablespoon almond butter
- Toppings: sliced banana, chia seeds, granola, berries

Instructions:

- In a blender, combine frozen banana, spinach, almond milk, and almond butter.
- Blend until smooth and creamy.
- Pour the smoothie into a bowl.
- Top with sliced banana, chia seeds, granola, and berries.

- Enjoy with a spoon.

Sweet Potato Hash:

Ingredients:

- 1 medium sweet potato, peeled and diced
- ½ onion, diced
- 1 bell pepper, diced
- 2 tablespoons olive oil
- Salt and pepper to taste
- Optional: smoked paprika, cayenne pepper, or other spices for flavor

Instructions:

- Heat olive oil in a skillet over medium heat.
- Add the diced sweet potato, onion, and bell pepper.
- Sauté until the sweet potato is cooked through and slightly crispy.
- Season with salt, pepper, and optional spices.
- Serve hot.

Yogurt and Fruit Smoothie:

Ingredients:

- 1 cup low-fat plain yogurt
- 1 cup mixed fresh or frozen fruit (banana, berries, mango, etc.)
- ½ cup unsweetened almond milk
- 1 tablespoon honey or maple syrup (optional)

Instructions:

- Place all the ingredients in a blender.
- Blend until smooth and creamy.
- Taste and add honey or maple syrup if desired.
- Pour into a glass and enjoy.

Almond Flour Pancakes:

Ingredients:

- 1 cup almond flour
- 2 eggs
- ¼ cup unsweetened almond milk
- 1 tablespoon honey or maple syrup
- ½ teaspoon baking powder
- ½ teaspoon vanilla extract
- Pinch of salt
- Cooking spray or butter for the pan

Instructions:

- In a bowl, whisk together almond flour, eggs, almond milk, honey/maple syrup, baking powder, vanilla extract, and salt until smooth.
- Heat a non-stick skillet over medium heat and coat with ay or butter.
- Pour about ¼ cup of the batter onto the skillet to form each pancake.
- Cook for 2-3 minutes on each side until golden brown.

- Repeat with the remaining batter.
- Serve with fresh fruit or sugar-free syrup.

Breakfast Quiche Cups:

Ingredients:

- 4 eggs
- ½ cup diced vegetables (spinach, mushrooms, onions, etc.)
- ¼ cup shredded low-fat cheese
- Salt and pepper to taste
- Cooking spray

Instructions:

- Preheat the oven to 350°F (175°C) and grease a muffin tin with cooking spray.
- In a bowl, whisk the eggs and season with salt and pepper.
- Stir in the diced vegetables and shredded cheese.
- Pour the mixture into the greased muffin tin, filling each cup about ¾ full.
- Bake for 15-20 minutes or until the quiche cups are set and golden.
- Remove from the oven, let cool slightly, and remove from the tin.
- Serve warm or refrigerate for later.

Whole Grain Toast with Almond Butter and Sliced Apples:

Ingredients:

- 1 slice whole grain bread
- 1 tablespoon almond butter
- ½ apple, thinly sliced
- Cinnamon for sprinkling

Instructions:

- Toast the bread until golden.
- Spread almond butter on the toast.
- Arrange the sliced apples on top.
- Sprinkle with cinnamon.
- Enjoy your delicious and simple toast.

Veggie Breakfast Burrito:

Ingredients:

- 1 whole wheat tortilla or wrap
- 2 eggs, scrambled
- ¼ cup diced mixed vegetables (bell peppers, onions, tomatoes, etc.)
- 2 tablespoons shredded low-fat cheese
- Salt and pepper to taste

Instructions:

- Heat a non-stick skillet over medium heat.
- Cook the scrambled eggs and diced vegetables together until the eggs are cooked through.

- Place the tortilla or wrap on a plate and layer the cooked eggs, shredded cheese, and seasoned vegetables in the center.
- Roll up the tortilla tightly, folding in the sides.
- Slice in half and enjoy.

20 gout-friendly lunch recipes, along with their ingredients and instructions, organized for you

LUNCH

Quinoa and Vegetable Stir-Fry

Ingredients:

- 1 cup cooked quinoa
- 1 cup mixed vegetables (broccoli, bell peppers, zucchini, carrots)
- 1 tablespoon low-sodium soy sauce
- 1 teaspoon sesame oil
- 1 clove garlic, minced

Instructions:

- In a pan, heat the sesame oil and sauté the minced garlic. Add the mixed vegetables and cook until tender. Stir in the cooked quinoa and soy sauce, and mix well.

Turkey and Avocado Wrap

Ingredients:

- 4 oz turkey slices
- 1 whole wheat tortilla
- 1/2 avocado, sliced
- Lettuce leaves
- Tomato slices
- Mustard or low-fat mayonnaise (optional)

Instructions:

- Lay the tortilla flat and layer turkey, avocado, lettuce, and tomato. Add mustard or mayo if desired. Roll it up tightly and cut in half.

Lentil Soup

Ingredients:

- 1 cup dried lentils
- 1 onion, chopped
- 2 carrots, diced
- 2 celery stalks, diced
- 4 cups low-sodium vegetable broth
- 1 teaspoon dried thyme
- Salt and pepper to taste

Instructions:

- In a pot, sauté the onions, carrots, and celery until softened. Add lentils, vegetable broth, thyme, salt, and pepper. Simmer until lentils are tender.

Baked Salmon with Steamed Asparagus

Ingredients:

- 6 oz salmon fillet
- Lemon slices
- Fresh dill (optional)
- 1 bunch asparagus
- Olive oil
- Salt and pepper to taste

Instructions:

- Preheat the oven to 375°F (190°C). Place the salmon on a baking sheet, season with salt, pepper, and dill, and top with lemon slices. Bake for 15-20 minutes. Meanwhile, steam the asparagus and drizzle with olive oil.

Spinach and Feta Stuffed Chicken Breast

Ingredients:

- 2 boneless, skinless chicken breasts
- 1 cup fresh spinach
- 1/4 cup crumbled feta cheese
- 1 clove garlic, minced
- Salt and pepper to taste

Instructions:

- Preheat the oven to 400°F (200°C). Butterfly the chicken breasts and stuff with spinach, feta, garlic, salt, and pepper. Secure with toothpicks and bake for 20-25 minutes.

Quinoa and Black Bean Salad

Ingredients:

- 1 cup cooked quinoa
- 1 can black beans, rinsed and drained
- 1 bell pepper, diced
- 1/4 cup chopped cilantro
- Lime juice
- Salt and cumin to taste

Instructions:

- In a bowl, combine quinoa, black beans, bell pepper, and cilantro. Squeeze lime juice over the salad and season with salt and cumin.

Greek Yogurt Chicken Wrap

Ingredients:

- 4 oz grilled chicken breast
- 1 whole wheat tortilla
- 2 tablespoons Greek yogurt
- 1 tablespoon hummus

- Cucumber slices
- Tomato slices
- Red onion slices
- Fresh parsley (optional)

Instructions:

- Spread Greek yogurt and hummus onto the tortilla. Layer grilled chicken, cucumber, tomato, onion, and parsley. Roll it up tightly and slice into rounds.

Vegetable Omelette

Ingredients:

- 3 eggs
- 1/4 cup diced bell peppers
- 1/4 cup diced onions
- 1/4 cup diced mushrooms
- 1/4 cup spinach leaves
- Salt and pepper to taste

Instructions:

- Whisk the eggs in a bowl and season with salt and pepper. In a non-stick pan, sauté the peppers, onions, mushrooms, and spinach. Pour the whisked eggs over the vegetables and cook until set.

Shrimp and Vegetable Skewers

Ingredients:

- 8 large shrimp, peeled and deveined
- Bell peppers, cut into chunks
- Red onion, cut into chunks
- Cherry tomatoes
- Olive oil
- Lemon juice
- Garlic powder
- Salt and pepper to taste

Instructions:

- Preheat the grill. Thread the shrimp, bell peppers, onion, and tomatoes onto skewers. Drizzle with olive oil, lemon juice, and sprinkle with garlic powder, salt, and pepper. Grill until shrimp are cooked through.

Zucchini Noodles with Tomato Sauce

Ingredients:

- 2 medium zucchinis, spiralized
- 1 cup tomato sauce (low-sodium)
- 1 clove garlic, minced
- 1 teaspoon olive oil
- Fresh basil leaves
- Salt and pepper to taste

Instructions:

- In a pan, heat olive oil and sauté minced garlic until fragrant. Add zucchini noodles and cook for 2-3 minutes. Pour in tomato sauce and cook until heated through. Season with salt and pepper. Garnish with fresh basil leaves.

Tuna Salad Lettuce Wraps

Ingredients:

- 1 can tuna, drained
- 2 tablespoons Greek yogurt
- 1 tablespoon lemon juice
- 1 celery stalk, diced
- 1/4 cup diced red onion
- Lettuce leaves
- Salt and pepper to taste

Instructions:

- In a bowl, mix tuna, Greek yogurt, lemon juice, celery, and red onion. Season with salt and pepper. Spoon the mixture onto lettuce leaves and wrap.

Tofu Stir-Fry with Brown Rice:

Ingredients:

- Extra-firm tofu, cubed
- Mixed vegetables (broccoli, carrots, snow peas)
- Garlic, minced
- Low-sodium soy sauce
- Sesame oil
- Ginger, grated
- Cooked brown rice

Instructions:

- Heat sesame oil in a skillet over medium heat.
- Add minced garlic and grated ginger, and sauté for a minute.
- Add cubed tofu and cook until lightly browned.
- Stir in mixed vegetables and cook until tender-crisp.
- Drizzle with low-sodium soy sauce and toss to coat.
- Serve over cooked brown rice.

Cucumber and Avocado Salad:

Ingredients:

- Cucumber, thinly sliced
- Avocado, diced
- Red onion, thinly sliced
- Fresh dill, chopped
- Lemon juice
- Olive oil
- Salt and pepper

Instructions:

- In a large bowl, combine thinly sliced cucumber, diced avocado, thinly sliced red onion, and chopped fresh dill.
- Drizzle with lemon juice and olive oil.
- Season with salt and pepper to taste.
- Toss gently to combine.
- Serve chilled.

Mediterranean Chicken Wrap:

Ingredients:

- Grilled chicken breast, sliced
- Whole wheat wrap or tortilla
- Hummus
- Cucumber, sliced
- Tomato, sliced
- Red onion, thinly sliced
- Kalamata olives, sliced
- Fresh parsley, chopped
- Lemon juice
- Salt and pepper

Instructions:

- Spread hummus evenly over the whole wheat wrap or tortilla.
- Layer grilled chicken slices, cucumber slices, tomato slices, thinly sliced red onion, and sliced kalamata olives.
- Sprinkle with fresh parsley.

- Drizzle with lemon juice.
- Season with salt and pepper to taste.
- Roll tightly to form a wrap.
- Cut in half and serve.

Egg Salad Lettuce Cups:

Ingredients:

- Hard-boiled eggs, peeled and chopped
- Greek yogurt (or mayonnaise)
- Dijon mustard
- Green onion, finely chopped
- Dill pickle, finely chopped
- Salt and pepper
- Lettuce leaves

Instructions:

- In a bowl, combine chopped hard-boiled eggs, Greek yogurt (or mayonnaise), Dijon mustard, finely chopped green onion, and finely chopped dill pickle.
- Season with salt and pepper to taste.
- Stir until well combined.
- Spoon the egg salad into lettuce leaves, forming cups.
- Serve chilled.

Cauliflower Fried Rice:

Ingredients:

- Cauliflower rice
- Mixed vegetables (carrots, peas, corn)
- Garlic, minced
- Low-sodium soy sauce
- Sesame oil
- Scrambled eggs (optional)
- Green onions, chopped

Instructions:

- Heat sesame oil in a skillet over medium heat.
- Add minced garlic and sauté until fragrant.
- Add mixed vegetables and cook until tender.
- Stir in cauliflower rice and cook until heated through.
- If desired, push the cauliflower rice mixture to one side of the skillet and scramble eggs on the other side.
- Once the eggs are cooked, mix everything together.
- Drizzle with low-sodium soy sauce and toss to coat.
- Stir in chopped green onions.
- Cook for a few more minutes until well combined.
- Serve hot.

Baked Cod with Roasted Vegetables:

Ingredients:

- Cod fillets
- Assorted vegetables (zucchini, bell peppers, cherry tomatoes)

- Garlic, minced
- Lemon juice
- Olive oil
- Dried herbs (such as thyme, rosemary, oregano)
- Salt and pepper

Instructions:

- Preheat oven to 400°F (200°C).
- Place cod fillets on a baking sheet lined with parchment paper.
- In a bowl, combine minced garlic, lemon juice, olive oil, dried herbs, salt, and pepper.
- Drizzle the mixture over the cod fillets.
- Toss assorted vegetables in the remaining mixture and place them around the cod on the baking sheet.
- Bake for 15-20 minutes or until the cod is cooked through and the vegetables are tender.
- Serve hot.

Chickpea Salad:

Ingredients:

- Canned chickpeas, drained and rinsed
- Cucumber, diced
- Cherry tomatoes, halved
- Red onion, diced
- Fresh parsley, chopped
- Lemon juice
- Olive oil
- Salt and pepper

Instructions:

- In a bowl, combine drained and rinsed chickpeas, diced cucumber, halved cherry tomatoes, diced red onion, and chopped fresh parsley.
- Drizzle with lemon juice and olive oil.
- Season with salt and pepper to taste.
- Toss gently to combine.
- Serve chilled.

Vegetable Omelette:

Ingredients:

- Eggs
- Bell peppers, diced
- Onion, diced
- Spinach leaves
- Low-fat cheese (optional)
- Salt and pepper
- Olive oil

Instructions:

- In a bowl, whisk eggs, salt, and pepper.
- Heat olive oil in a non-stick skillet over medium heat.
- Sauté diced bell peppers and onions until softened.
- Add spinach leaves and cook until wilted.
- Pour the beaten eggs over the vegetables in the skillet.
- Cook until the omelette is set.

- Sprinkle with low-fat cheese (optional) and fold in half.
- Cook for another minute until the cheese melts.

- Serve hot.

Shrimp Stir-Fry with Brown Rice:

Ingredients:

- Shrimp, peeled and deveined
- Mixed vegetables (broccoli, bell peppers, snap peas)
- Garlic, minced
- Low-sodium soy sauce
- Sesame oil
- Cooked brown rice

Instructions:

- Heat sesame oil in a skillet over medium heat.
- Add minced garlic and sauté until fragrant.
- Add shrimp and cook until they turn pink.
- Stir in the mixed vegetables and cook until tender-crisp.
- Drizzle with low-sodium soy sauce and toss to coat.
- Serve over cooked brown rice.

Greek Salad with Grilled Chicken:

Ingredients:

- Grilled chicken breast, sliced
- Cucumber, diced
- Cherry tomatoes, halved
- Kalamata olives
- Red onion, thinly sliced
- Feta cheese, crumbled

- Lemon juice
- Extra-virgin olive oil
- Dried oregano
- Salt and pepper

Instructions:

- In a large bowl, combine cucumber, cherry tomatoes, kalamata olives, and thinly sliced red onion.
- Top with sliced grilled chicken breast and crumbled feta cheese.
- Drizzle with lemon juice and extra-virgin olive oil.
- Sprinkle with dried oregano, salt, and pepper.
- Toss gently to combine.
- Serve chilled.

Black Bean and Corn Salad:

Ingredients:

- Canned black beans, drained and rinsed
- Corn kernels (fresh or canned), drained
- Red bell pepper, diced
- Red onion, diced
- Cilantro, chopped
- Lime juice
- Olive oil
- Cumin
- Salt and pepper

Instructions:

- In a large bowl, combine black beans, corn kernels, diced red bell pepper, diced red onion, and chopped cilantro.
- Drizzle with lime juice and olive oil.
- Sprinkle with cumin, salt, and pepper.
- Toss gently to combine.
- Refrigerate for at least 30 minutes before serving.
- Serve chilled.

Enjoy your gout diet dinner recipes!

DINNER

Quinoa Stuffed Bell Peppers:

Ingredients:

- 4 bell peppers
- 1 cup cooked quinoa
- 1 can black beans, drained and rinsed
- 1 cup diced tomatoes
- 1 cup diced zucchini
- 1 cup diced onions
- 1 teaspoon cumin
- Salt and pepper to taste

Instructions:

- Preheat oven to 375°F (190°C).
- Cut the tops off the bell peppers and remove the seeds.

- In a bowl, mix cooked quinoa, black beans, diced tomatoes, zucchini, onions, cumin, salt, and pepper.
- Stuff the bell peppers with the quinoa mixture.
- Place the stuffed bell peppers in a baking dish and bake for 25-30 minutes or until the peppers are tender.

Turkey Lettuce Wraps:

Ingredients:

- 1 pound ground turkey
- 1 tablespoon olive oil
- 2 cloves garlic, minced
- 1 teaspoon ginger, grated
- 1 tablespoon low-sodium soy sauce
- 1 tablespoon rice vinegar
- 1 tablespoon honey
- 1 cup shredded carrots
- 1 cup sliced mushrooms
- 8 large lettuce leaves

Instructions:

- Heat olive oil in a skillet over medium heat.
- Add ground turkey, garlic, and ginger to the skillet. Cook until turkey is browned and cooked through.
- In a small bowl, mix soy sauce, rice vinegar, and honey.
- Add the sauce, shredded carrots, and mushrooms to the skillet. Cook for another 2-3 minutes.
- Spoon the turkey mixture into lettuce leaves and serve.

Grilled Shrimp Skewers:

Ingredients:

- 1 pound shrimp, peeled and deveined
- 2 tablespoons olive oil
- 2 cloves garlic, minced
- 1 teaspoon paprika
- 1/2 teaspoon cayenne pepper
- Salt and pepper to taste
- Instructions:
- Preheat grill to medium-high heat.
- In a bowl, mix olive oil, garlic, paprika, cayenne pepper, salt, and pepper.
- Add shrimp to the mixture and toss to coat.
- Thread shrimp onto skewers and grill for 2-3 minutes per side or until shrimp is pink and cooked through.
- Serve with a side of brown rice and steamed asparagus.

Lentil Vegetable Soup:

Ingredients:

- 1 cup green lentils, rinsed
- 1 cup chopped carrots
- 1 cup chopped celery
- 1 cup diced tomatoes
- 1 cup chopped onions
- 2 cloves garlic, minced
- 4 cups vegetable broth
- 1 teaspoon dried thyme
- Salt and pepper to taste

Instructions:

- In a large pot, combine lentils, carrots, celery, tomatoes, onions, garlic, vegetable broth, thyme, salt, and pepper.
- Bring the mixture to a boil, then reduce heat and simmer for about 30 minutes or until the lentils are tender.
- Adjust seasoning if needed.
- Serve hot.

Grilled Steak with Roasted Potatoes:

Ingredients:

- 4 beef steaks (sirloin, strip, or ribeye)
- 1 pound baby potatoes, halved
- 2 tablespoons olive oil
- 2 cloves garlic, minced
- 1 teaspoon dried rosemary
- Salt and pepper to taste

Instructions:

- Preheat grill to medium-high heat.
- In a bowl, mix olive oil, garlic, rosemary, salt, and pepper.
- Toss the halved potatoes with the olive oil mixture and spread them on a baking sheet.
- Roast the potatoes in the oven at 400°F (200°C) for about 20-25 minutes or until golden brown and tender.
- Season the steaks with salt and pepper, then grill for 4-5 minutes per side or until desired doneness.

- Serve the grilled steaks with roasted potatoes.

Baked Chicken and Vegetables:

Ingredients:

- 4 bone-in, skin-on chicken thighs
- 2 tablespoons olive oil
- 1 teaspoon dried oregano
- 1 teaspoon dried thyme
- 1 teaspoon paprika
- Salt and pepper to taste
- 1 pound mixed vegetables (carrots, broccoli, cauliflower)
- Instructions:
- Preheat oven to 400°F (200°C).
- Rub chicken thighs with olive oil, oregano, thyme, paprika, salt, and pepper.
- Place chicken thighs in a baking dish.
- Toss the mixed vegetables with olive oil, salt, and pepper.
- Spread the vegetables around the chicken thighs.
- Bake for 30-35 minutes or until the chicken is cooked through and the vegetables are tender.

Tofu Stir-Fry:

Ingredients:

- 1 block firm tofu, drained and cubed
- 2 tablespoons low-sodium soy sauce

- 1 tablespoon rice vinegar
- 1 tablespoon honey
- 2 tablespoons sesame oil
- 2 cloves garlic, minced
- 1 teaspoon grated ginger
- 2 cups mixed stir-fry vegetables (broccoli, bell peppers, snap peas)
- Salt and pepper to taste

Instructions:

- In a bowl, mix soy sauce, rice vinegar, honey, sesame oil, garlic, ginger, salt, and pepper.
- Add tofu cubes to the sauce and let marinate for 15 minutes.
- Heat a skillet or wok over medium heat and add the marinated tofu with the sauce.
- Cook for about 5 minutes until tofu is browned.
- Add the mixed stir-fry vegetables to the skillet and cook for another 3-4 minutes until vegetables are tender.
- Serve over steamed brown rice.

Roasted Cauliflower Steaks:

Ingredients:

- 1 head cauliflower
- 2 tablespoons olive oil
- 1 teaspoon smoked paprika
- 1/2 teaspoon garlic powder
- Salt and pepper to taste

Instructions:

- Preheat oven to 425°F (220°C).
- Remove the leaves from the cauliflower and trim the stem, leaving the core intact.
- Slice the cauliflower into 1-inch thick steaks.
- In a bowl, mix olive oil, smoked paprika, garlic powder, salt, and pepper.
- Brush both sides of the cauliflower steaks with the olive oil mixture.
- Place the cauliflower steaks on a baking sheet and roast for 20-25 minutes, flipping halfway through, or until the cauliflower is tender and browned.
- Serve as a main dish or as a side with a green salad.

Greek Salad with Grilled Chicken:

Ingredients:

- 2 boneless, skinless chicken breasts
- 4 cups mixed salad greens
- 1 cup cherry tomatoes, halved
- 1 cucumber, diced
- 1/2 red onion, thinly sliced
- 1/2 cup Kalamata olives, pitted
- 1/2 cup crumbled feta cheese
- 2 tablespoons olive oil
- 1 tablespoon red wine vinegar
- 1 teaspoon dried oregano
- Salt and pepper to taste

Instructions:

- Preheat grill to medium-high heat.
- Season chicken breasts with salt, pepper, and dried oregano.
- Grill chicken for about 6-8 minutes per side or until cooked through.
- Let the chicken rest for a few minutes, then slice it into thin strips.
- In a large bowl, combine salad greens, cherry tomatoes, cucumber, red onion, Kalamata olives, and feta cheese.
- In a small bowl, whisk together olive oil, red wine vinegar, dried oregano, salt, and pepper.
- Drizzle the dressing over the salad and toss to coat.
- Top the salad with grilled chicken slices.

Eggplant Parmesan:

Ingredients:

- 2 medium eggplants, sliced into 1/2-inch rounds
- 2 cups marinara sauce
- 1 cup shredded mozzarella cheese
- 1/2 cup grated Parmesan cheese
- 1/2 cup breadcrumbs
- 2 tablespoons olive oil
- 2 tablespoons chopped fresh basil
- Salt and pepper to taste

- Preheat oven to 375°F (190°C).
- Sprinkle salt on both sides of the eggplant slices and let them sit for 15 minutes to remove excess moisture.
- Rinse the eggplant slices and pat them dry.
- In a shallow dish, combine breadcrumbs, grated Parmesan cheese, salt, and pepper.
- Dip each eggplant slice in the breadcrumb mixture, coating both sides.
- Heat olive oil in a skillet over medium heat.
- Cook the breaded eggplant slices for 2-3 minutes per side or until golden brown.
- In a baking dish, spread a thin layer of marinara sauce.
- Arrange half of the cooked eggplant slices on top of the sauce.
- Sprinkle half of the mozzarella cheese and basil over the eggplant.
- Repeat the layers with the remaining ingredients.
- Bake for 20-25 minutes or until the cheese is melted and bubbly.
- Serve with a side of whole wheat spaghetti.

Seared Tuna with Quinoa Salad:

Ingredients:

- 2 tuna steaks
- 1 cup cooked quinoa
- 1 cup diced cucumbers
- 1 cup cherry tomatoes, halved

- 1/2 cup diced red bell pepper
- 1/4 cup chopped fresh parsley
- 2 tablespoons lemon juice
- 2 tablespoons olive oil
- Salt and pepper to taste

Instructions:

- Season tuna steaks with salt and pepper.
- Heat a skillet or grill pan over high heat.
- Sear the tuna steaks for 2-3 minutes per side or until desired doneness.
- In a large bowl, combine cooked quinoa, cucumbers, cherry tomatoes, red bell pepper, parsley, lemon juice, olive oil, salt, and pepper. Toss to combine.
- Slice the seared tuna and serve over the quinoa salad.

Stir-Fried Beef with Broccoli:

Ingredients:

- 1 pound beef sirloin, thinly sliced
- 2 tablespoons low-sodium soy sauce
- 1 tablespoon cornstarch
- 1 tablespoon olive oil
- 2 cloves garlic, minced
- 1 teaspoon grated ginger
- 2 cups broccoli florets
- 1/2 cup beef broth
- 1 tablespoon oyster sauce

Salt and pepper to taste

Instructions:

- In a bowl, mix soy sauce and cornstarch. Add the sliced beef and toss to coat. Let it marinate for 15 minutes.
- Heat olive oil in a skillet or wok over medium-high heat.
- Add garlic and ginger to the skillet and cook for 1 minute.
- Add the marinated beef to the skillet and stir-fry for about 3-4 minutes or until browned.
- Add broccoli florets, beef broth, oyster sauce, salt, and pepper to the skillet.
- Stir-fry for another 3-4 minutes or until the broccoli is crisp-tender and the beef is cooked through.
- Serve over cooked brown rice.

Quinoa Stuffed Bell Peppers:

- **Ingredients:**
- 4 bell peppers (any color), tops removed and seeded
- 1 cup cooked quinoa
- 1 cup canned black beans, rinsed and drained
- 1 cup corn kernels
- 1/2 cup diced tomatoes
- 1/2 cup shredded cheddar cheese
- 2 tablespoons chopped fresh cilantro
- 1 tablespoon olive oil
- 1 teaspoon ground cumin
- Salt and pepper to taste

Instructions:

- Preheat oven to 375°F (190°C).
- In a large bowl, combine cooked quinoa, black beans, corn kernels, diced tomatoes, shredded cheddar cheese, chopped cilantro, olive oil, ground cumin, salt, and pepper.
- Stuff each bell pepper with the quinoa mixture.
- Place the stuffed bell peppers in a baking dish and cover with foil.
- Bake for 25-30 minutes or until the peppers are tender.
- Remove the foil and bake for an additional 5 minutes to melt the cheese.
- Serve hot.

Salmon with Dill Sauce:

Ingredients:

- 4 salmon fillets
- 2 tablespoons lemon juice
- 2 tablespoons melted butter
- 1 tablespoon chopped fresh dill
- 1 tablespoon Dijon mustard
- Salt and pepper to taste

Instructions:

- Preheat oven to 400°F (200°C).
- Season salmon fillets with salt and pepper.
- In a small bowl, mix lemon juice, melted butter, chopped dill, and Dijon mustard.

- Place the salmon fillets on a baking sheet lined with parchment paper.
- Brush the lemon and dill sauce over the salmon fillets, coating them evenly.
- Bake for 12-15 minutes or until the salmon is cooked through and flakes easily with a fork.
- Serve with a side of steamed asparagus or roasted vegetables.

Quinoa and Vegetable Stir-Fry:

Ingredients:

- 1 cup cooked quinoa
- 1 tablespoon olive oil
- 1 cup sliced mushrooms
- 1 cup sliced bell peppers (any color)
- 1 cup snow peas
- 1 cup sliced zucchini
- 2 cloves garlic, minced
- 2 tablespoons low-sodium soy sauce
- 1 tablespoon sesame oil
- Salt and pepper to taste

Instructions:

- Heat olive oil in a skillet or wok over medium-high heat.
- Add mushrooms, bell peppers, snow peas, and zucchini to the skillet and stir-fry for about 3-4 minutes or until vegetables are crisp-tender.
- Add minced garlic to the skillet and cook for an additional minute.

- Add cooked quinoa, soy sauce, sesame oil, salt, and pepper to the skillet. Stir-fry for another 2-3 minutes to heat everything through.
- Serve hot.

DESSERTS

Grilled Pineapple with Coconut Yogurt

Ingredients:

- 1 fresh pineapple (sliced)
- 1 cup Greek yogurt (unsweetened)
- 2 tbsp shredded coconut

Instructions:

- Grill the pineapple slices for a few minutes on each side.
- Serve with a dollop of Greek yogurt and sprinkle shredded coconut on top.

Raspberry Chia Jam

Ingredients:

- 2 cups raspberries
- 2 tbsp chia seeds
- 2 tbsp honey

Instructions:

- Blend the raspberries until smooth.

- Mix in chia seeds and honey.
- Refrigerate for 1-2 hours to thicken.

Peach and Almond Crumble

Ingredients:

- 4 ripe peaches (sliced)
- 1/2 cup almond flour
- 2 tbsp honey
- 1/4 tsp cinnamon
- 2 tbsp unsalted butter (melted)

Instructions:

- Preheat the oven to 375°F (190°C).
- Mix almond flour, honey, cinnamon, and melted butter to form the crumble.
- Arrange the peach slices in a baking dish and top with the crumble.
- Bake for 25-30 minutes until golden brown.

Lemon Basil Sorbet

Ingredients:

- 1 cup fresh lemon juice
- 1/4 cup honey
- 1/4 cup fresh basil leaves (chopped)
- 1 cup water

Instructions:

- Combine lemon juice, honey, basil, and water in a blender.
- Blend until smooth.
- Pour the mixture into a shallow dish and freeze for at least 4 hours.

Coconut Macaroons

Ingredients:

- 2 cups unsweetened shredded coconut
- 3 egg whites
- 1/4 cup honey
- 1/2 tsp vanilla extract

Instructions:

- Preheat the oven to 325°F (165°C).
- Mix shredded coconut, egg whites, honey, and vanilla extract in a bowl.
- Drop spoonfuls of the mixture onto a baking sheet lined with parchment paper.
- Bake for 20-25 minutes until golden brown.

Greek Yogurt Parfait

Ingredients:

- 1 cup Greek yogurt (unsweetened)
- 1/2 cup mixed berries
- 2 tbsp chopped nuts (e.g., almonds, walnuts)
- 1 tbsp honey
- Instructions:
- Layer Greek yogurt, mixed berries, and chopped nuts in a glass or bowl.

- Drizzle honey on top and serve.

Strawberry Banana Smoothie

Ingredients:

- 1 cup frozen strawberries
- 1 ripe banana
- 1 cup unsweetened almond milk
- 1 tbsp honey
- Instructions:
- Blend all the ingredients until smooth.

Cantaloupe and Prosciutto Skewers

Ingredients:

- 1/2 cantaloupe (cut into bite-sized cubes)
- 8 thin slices of prosciutto
- Wooden skewers

Instructions:

- Wrap each cantaloupe cube with a slice of prosciutto and thread onto a skewer.

Baked Pears with Honey and Cinnamon

Ingredients:

- 4 ripe pears
- 2 tbsp honey
- 1 tsp ground cinnamon

Instructions:

- Preheat the oven to 375°F (190°C).
- Cut pears in half and remove the cores.
- Place the pear halves on a baking sheet.
- Drizzle honey and sprinkle cinnamon over the pears.
- Bake for 25-30 minutes until tender.

Frozen Yogurt Bark

Ingredients:

- 2 cups Greek yogurt (unsweetened)
- 1/4 cup honey
- 1/2 cup mixed berries (chopped)
- 2 tbsp unsalted nuts (e.g., almonds, pistachios)
- Instructions:
- Mix Greek yogurt and honey in a bowl.
- Spread the mixture onto a parchment-lined baking sheet.
- Sprinkle chopped berries and nuts on top.
- Freeze for 2-3 hours until firm, then break into pieces.

Mango Sorbet

Ingredients:

- 2 ripe mangoes (peeled and cubed)

- 2 tbsp lime juice
- 2 tbsp honey
- 1/2 cup water
- Instructions:
- Blend mangoes, lime juice, honey, and water until smooth.
- Pour the mixture into a shallow dish and freeze for at least 4 hours.

Peanut Butter Banana Bites

Ingredients:

- 2 ripe bananas
- 2 tbsp natural peanut butter
- 1/4 cup crushed peanuts
- Instructions:
- Peel the bananas and slice them into rounds.
- Spread peanut butter on half of the banana rounds.
- Sandwich them with the other banana rounds.
- Roll the edges in crushed peanuts.

Mixed Fruit Salad

Ingredients:

- 1 cup diced pineapple
- 1 cup diced watermelon
- 1 cup grapes
- 1 cup diced kiwi
- Juice of 1 lime

- Instructions:
- Combine all the fruits in a bowl.
- Squeeze lime juice over the fruit and toss gently.

Chia Seed Pudding:

Ingredients:

- 1 cup unsweetened almond milk
- 3 tablespoons chia seeds
- 1 tablespoon honey
- 1/2 teaspoon vanilla extract
- Fresh berries for topping

Instructions:

- In a bowl, mix the almond milk, chia seeds, honey, and vanilla extract.
- Stir well to combine.
- Cover the bowl and refrigerate overnight or for at least 2 hours until the mixture thickens.
- Stir the pudding before serving and top with fresh berries.

Greek Yogurt with Nuts and Honey:

Ingredients:

- 1 cup low-fat Greek yogurt
- 2 tablespoons chopped mixed nuts (almonds, pistachios, walnuts)

- 1 tablespoon honey
- Instructions:
- In a bowl, add the Greek yogurt.
- Sprinkle the chopped mixed nuts over the yogurt.
- Drizzle honey over the top.
- Mix well and enjoy.

Watermelon Granita:

Ingredients:

- 4 cups cubed seedless watermelon
- Juice of 1 lime
- 2 tablespoons honey
- Fresh mint leaves for garnish

Instructions:

- In a blender, combine the watermelon, lime juice, and honey.
- Blend until smooth.
- Pour the mixture into a shallow dish.
- Place in the freezer for 1 hour.
- After 1 hour, scrape the mixture with a fork to break up any ice crystals.
- Repeat this process every 30 minutes for about 3 hours or until the mixture has a slushy consistency.
- Serve in bowls or glasses and garnish with fresh mint leaves.

Almond Butter Banana Bites:

Ingredients:

- 2 ripe bananas
- 2 tablespoons almond butter
- 2 tablespoons unsweetened shredded coconut
- Instructions:
- Peel the bananas and slice them into 1-inch thick rounds.
- Spread a small amount of almond butter on top of each banana slice.
- Sprinkle shredded coconut over the almond butter.
- Place the banana bites on a plate and freeze for at least 1 hour.
- Serve chilled.

Avocado Chocolate Mousse:

Ingredients:

- 2 ripe avocados
- 1/4 cup unsweetened cocoa powder
- 1/4 cup honey or maple syrup
- 1 teaspoon vanilla extract
- Fresh berries for topping (optional)
- Instructions:
- Cut the avocados in half, remove the pits, and scoop out the flesh.
- In a blender or food processor, combine the avocado flesh, cocoa powder, honey or maple syrup, and vanilla extract.

- Blend until smooth and creamy.
- Spoon the mousse into serving dishes.
- Refrigerate for at least 1 hour.
- Top with fresh berries before serving.

Yogurt Bark:

Ingredients:

- 1 cup low-fat Greek yogurt
- 1 tablespoon honey
- 1/4 cup chopped mixed nuts (almonds, pistachios, walnuts)
- 1/4 cup fresh berries

Instructions:

- Line a baking sheet with parchment paper.
- In a bowl, mix the Greek yogurt and honey.
- Spread the yogurt mixture evenly on the prepared baking sheet.
- Sprinkle the chopped mixed nuts and fresh berries over the yogurt.
- Place the baking sheet in the freezer for 2-3 hours until the yogurt is firm.
- Break the yogurt bark into pieces and serve.

Grilled Pineapple:

Ingredients:

- 1 pineapple, peeled and cored

- 1 tablespoon honey
- Ground cinnamon (optional)
- Instructions:
- Preheat the grill to medium heat.
- Slice the pineapple into rings or spears.
- Brush each pineapple slice with honey.
- Grill the pineapple for 2-3 minutes per side until it has grill marks and is slightly caramelized.
- Sprinkle with ground cinnamon if desired.
- Serve warm.

Lemon Bars:

Ingredients:

- 1 cup almond flour
- 1/4 cup coconut flour
- 1/4 cup melted coconut oil
- 1/4 cup fresh lemon juice
- Zest of 1 lemon
- 3 eggs
- 1/4 cup honey or maple syrup
- 1/4 teaspoon baking soda

Instructions:

- Preheat the oven to 350°F (175°C) and line a baking dish with parchment paper.
- In a bowl, mix the almond flour, coconut flour, melted coconut oil, and baking soda until well combined.
- Press the mixture into the bottom of the prepared baking dish to form the crust.

- In another bowl, whisk together the fresh lemon juice, lemon zest, eggs, and honey or maple syrup.
- Pour the lemon mixture over the crust.
- Bake for 20-25 minutes or until the edges are golden brown and the center is set.
- Allow the bars to cool completely before cutting into squares.

SNACKS

Here are 20 gout-friendly snack recipes along with their ingredients and instructions:

Almond and Blueberry Smoothie:

Ingredients:

- 1 cup almond milk
- 1/2 cup blueberries
- 1 tablespoon almond butter
- 1 tablespoon honey (optional)
- Ice cubes (optional)

Instructions:

- In a blender, combine the almond milk, blueberries, almond butter, and honey.
- Blend until smooth and creamy.
- Add ice cubes if desired and blend again.
- Pour into a glass and enjoy.

Quinoa Salad Cups:

Ingredients:

- 1 cup cooked quinoa
- 1/2 cup cucumber, diced
- 1/2 cup cherry tomatoes, halved
- 1/4 cup feta cheese, crumbled
- 2 tablespoons fresh lemon juice
- 1 tablespoon olive oil
- Salt and pepper to taste
- Fresh mint leaves for garnish

Instructions:

- In a bowl, combine the cooked quinoa, diced cucumber, cherry tomatoes, and crumbled feta cheese.
- In a separate small bowl, whisk together the lemon juice, olive oil, salt, and pepper.
- Pour the dressing over the quinoa mixture and toss gently to combine.
- Spoon the salad into small cups or lettuce wraps.
- Garnish with fresh mint leaves and serve.

Spinach and Feta Stuffed Mushrooms:

Ingredients:

- 8 large mushrooms
- 2 cups fresh spinach, chopped
- 1/4 cup feta cheese, crumbled
- 2 cloves garlic, minced
- 1 tablespoon olive oil

- Salt and pepper to taste

Instructions:

- Preheat the oven to 375°F (190°C).
- Remove the stems from the mushrooms and set aside.
- In a pan, heat the olive oil over medium heat and sauté the mushroom stems, spinach, and garlic until the spinach wilts.
- Season with salt and pepper.
- Stuff the mushroom caps with the spinach mixture and place them on a baking sheet.
- Sprinkle feta cheese on top of each mushroom.
- Bake for 15-20 minutes until the mushrooms are tender and the cheese is melted.
- Let cool slightly before serving.

Greek Salad Skewers:

Ingredients:

- 1 cup cherry tomatoes
- 1 cup cucumber, diced
- 1/2 cup black olives
- 1/2 cup feta cheese, cubed
- 2 tablespoons olive oil
- 1 tablespoon fresh lemon juice
- 1 teaspoon dried oregano
- Salt and pepper to taste
- Wooden skewers

Instructions:

- Thread cherry tomatoes, cucumber, black olives, and feta cheese alternately onto wooden skewers.
- In a small bowl, whisk together olive oil, lemon juice, dried oregano, salt, and pepper to make the dressing.
- Drizzle the dressing over the skewers.
- Serve as a delicious and colorful appetizer.

Tuna Lettuce Wraps:

Ingredients:

- 1 can tuna, drained
- 1/4 cup celery, diced
- 1/4 cup red onion, finely chopped
- 2 tablespoons mayonnaise
- 1 tablespoon Dijon mustard
- Salt and pepper to taste
- Lettuce leaves for wrapping

Instructions:

- In a bowl, combine the tuna, celery, red onion, mayonnaise, Dijon mustard, salt, and pepper.
- Mix well until all ingredients are well combined.
- Spoon the tuna mixture onto lettuce leaves and wrap them up.
- Secure with toothpicks if needed and enjoy.

Egg and Vegetable Muffins:

Ingredients:

- 6 eggs
- 1/2 cup bell peppers, diced
- 1/2 cup zucchini, grated
- 1/4 cup onion, finely chopped
- 1/4 cup feta cheese, crumbled
- Salt and pepper to taste

Instructions:

- Preheat the oven to 350°F (175°C) and grease a muffin tin.
- In a bowl, whisk the eggs and season with salt and pepper.
- Add the diced bell peppers, grated zucchini, chopped onion, and crumbled feta cheese to the egg mixture. Stir to combine.
- Pour the mixture evenly into the greased muffin tin.
- Bake for 20-25 minutes or until the muffins are set and lightly golden.
- Allow them to cool slightly before removing from the tin.
- Serve as individual egg muffins.

Greek Yogurt and Berry Parfait:

Ingredients:

- 1 cup Greek yogurt
- 1/2 cup mixed berries (blueberries, strawberries, raspberries)
- 2 tablespoons honey
- 2 tablespoons granola (optional)

Instructions:

- In a glass or bowl, layer Greek yogurt, mixed berries, and honey.
- Repeat the layers until all ingredients are used.
- Top with granola for added crunch, if desired.
- Serve chilled as a healthy and satisfying snack

14-Days Meal Plan for Endometriosis Diet

Here is a 14-day meal plan for an endometriosis diet cookbook. I can assist you in developing a comprehensive 14-day meal plan that is gout-friendly as a dietitian. High uric acid levels in the blood cause gout, a kind of arthritis, and specific foods can worsen or start an attack. An anti-inflammatory diet for gout aims to control uric acid levels. To get you started, here is an example meal schedule:

Day 1:

Breakfast: Oatmeal topped with fresh berries and a sprinkle of chopped almonds. Serve with a cup of green tea.

Snack: Carrot sticks with hummus.

Lunch: Grilled chicken breast salad with mixed greens, cherry tomatoes, cucumbers, and a lemon vinaigrette dressing.

Snack: Greek yogurt with a handful of walnuts.

Dinner: Baked salmon with roasted asparagus and quinoa.

Dessert: Sliced melon.

Day 2:

Breakfast: Vegetable omelet made with egg whites, spinach, bell peppers, and mushrooms. Serve with a slice of whole-grain toast.

Snack: Celery sticks with almond butter.

Lunch: Quinoa salad with diced chicken breast, black beans, cherry tomatoes, and avocado.

Snack: A handful of grapes.

Dinner: Grilled shrimp skewers with zucchini noodles and a side of steamed broccoli.

Dessert: Sugar-free gelatin.

Day 3:

Breakfast: Whole-grain toast with mashed avocado and sliced tomatoes. Enjoy with a cup of herbal tea.

Snack: Sliced cucumbers with tzatziki sauce.

Lunch: Lentil soup with a side of mixed greens salad.

Snack: Apple slices with a tablespoon of peanut butter.

Dinner: Grilled chicken breast with roasted Brussels sprouts and quinoa.

Dessert: Mixed berries with a dollop of Greek yogurt.

Day 4:

Breakfast: Overnight chia pudding made with almond milk, chia seeds, and fresh fruit.

Snack: Hard-boiled eggs.

Lunch: Spinach salad with grilled tofu, cherry tomatoes, cucumbers, and a balsamic vinaigrette dressing.

Snack: Edamame.

Dinner: Baked cod with steamed green beans and brown rice.

Dessert: A small handful of almonds.

Day 5 :

Breakfast: Quinoa porridge with mixed berries and almond milk.

Snack: A handful of unsalted almonds.

Lunch: Grilled chicken breast salad with mixed greens, cherry tomatoes, cucumber, and balsamic vinaigrette.

Snack: Greek yogurt with diced pineapple.

Dinner: Baked salmon with steamed asparagus and quinoa.

Evening snack: Carrot sticks with hummus.

Day 6 :

Breakfast: Oatmeal topped with sliced bananas and a drizzle of honey.

Snack: Celery sticks with almond butter.

Lunch: Quinoa salad with diced chicken breast, bell peppers, cherry tomatoes, and lemon vinaigrette.

Snack: Mixed berries with a dollop of Greek yogurt.

Dinner: Grilled lean steak with roasted sweet potatoes and steamed broccoli.

Evening snack: Sliced cucumbers with tzatziki dip.

Day 7 :

Breakfast: Vegetable omelet with spinach, mushrooms, and bell peppers.

Snack: A handful of walnuts.

Lunch: Lentil soup with a side of mixed greens salad.

Snack: Sliced apples with a sprinkle of cinnamon.

Dinner: Baked cod with quinoa pilaf and roasted Brussels sprouts.

Evening snack: Sugar snap peas with hummus.

Continue with a similar pattern for the following days:

Day 8 :

Breakfast: Greek yogurt with sliced peaches and a sprinkle of chia seeds.

Snack: Hard-boiled eggs.

Lunch: Quinoa-stuffed bell peppers with a side of mixed greens.

Snack: Cherry tomatoes with mozzarella cheese.

Dinner: Grilled shrimp skewers with brown rice and grilled zucchini.

Evening snack: Edamame beans.

Day 9 :

Breakfast: Whole grain toast with avocado and poached eggs.

Snack: Cottage cheese with sliced cucumbers.

Lunch: Chicken and vegetable stir-fry with brown rice.

Snack: Mixed fruit salad.

Dinner: Grilled chicken breast with roasted cauliflower and quinoa.

Evening snack: Rice cakes with almond butter.

Day 10:

Breakfast: Overnight chia pudding with almond milk, topped with sliced bananas and chopped walnuts.

Lunch: Chickpea salad with diced tomatoes, cucumbers, parsley, and lemon dressing.

Snack: Rice cakes with almond butter.

Dinner: Turkey chili with kidney beans and a side of steamed green beans.

Snack: Mixed berries.

Day 11:

Breakfast: Vegetable and egg scramble with whole wheat tortilla.

Lunch: Grilled chicken Caesar salad with romaine lettuce, cherry tomatoes, and light Caesar dressing.

Snack: Homemade trail mix (unsalted nuts, dried fruit, and seeds).

Dinner: Baked tofu with stir-fried mixed vegetables and brown rice.

Snack: Sliced bell peppers with guacamole.

Day 12:

Breakfast: Smoothie made with almond milk, spinach, frozen berries, and a scoop of protein powder.

Lunch: Quinoa-stuffed bell peppers with black beans, corn, and diced tomatoes.

Snack: Cottage cheese with pineapple chunks.

Dinner: Grilled salmon with roasted zucchini and wild rice.

Snack: Grapes.

Day 13:

Breakfast: Smoothie made with almond milk, spinach, banana, and a scoop of protein powder

Hard-boiled egg

Lunch: Caprese salad with tomatoes, fresh mozzarella, and basil

Whole-grain crackers

Snack: Orange slices

Dinner: Grilled chicken skewers with bell peppers and onions

Brown rice

Grilled asparagus

Day 14:

Breakfast:Whole-grain toast topped with mashed avocado and sliced tomatoes

Boiled egg

Lunch:Grilled vegetable wrap with whole-wheat tortilla, hummus, and feta cheese

Snack:Celery sticks with peanut butter

Dinner:Baked chicken breast

Quinoa with roasted vegetables

Steamed Brussels sprouts

In conclusion, this cookbook offers a wealth of practical information, delicious recipes, and a structured meal plan to help individuals successfully navigate the challenges of gout management. By embracing the principles outlined in this book, readers can take proactive steps towards improved health and well-being, making "The New Healthy Recipes Gout Diet Cookbook Bible" an invaluable companion on their journey to a healthier life.

In conclusion, "The New Healthy Recipes Gout Diet Cookbook Bible" is a comprehensive guide that empowers individuals to take control of their health and manage gout through delicious and nutritious meals. With a collection of 100 carefully crafted recipes and a well-structured 14-day meal plan, this cookbook serves as a valuable resource for those seeking a healthier lifestyle while dealing with gout.

Throughout the book, readers are introduced to a wide variety of flavorful dishes that prioritize ingredients known to alleviate gout symptoms and promote overall well-being. The recipes emphasize the use of fresh, whole foods, incorporating a balanced combination of lean proteins, colorful fruits and vegetables, and whole grains.

By following the provided 14-day meal plan, readers can simplify their journey towards healthier eating habits. The plan offers a clear roadmap, allowing individuals to effortlessly navigate their dietary choices and make positive changes to their daily routine. The inclusion of a meal plan not only ensures a well-rounded nutritional intake but also adds convenience and peace of mind for those looking to make sustainable dietary changes.

"The New Healthy Recipes Gout Diet Cookbook Bible" goes beyond just providing recipes and meal plans. It also educates readers on the principles of gout management, highlighting the importance of hydration, regular exercise, and portion control. The book serves as an all-in-one resource, equipping readers with the knowledge and tools needed to make informed decisions about their diet and overall lifestyle. Gout can often be successfully treated and managed. Your doctor may prescribe medications that help lower your uric acid levels and reduce inflammation and pain.

Your doctor or nutritionist can also recommend changes in your diet to help prevent flare-ups. Balanced eating and healthy lifestyle habits can help you successfully manage gout.

Always check with your doctor first before adding a supplement to your regimen. Interactions and side effects could be possible with herbal supplements.

Never replace your established, prescribed gout treatments with a home remedy without informing your doctor. None of the herbal supplements recommended are regulated by the U.S. Food and Drug Administration for what they contain or how well they work. Only purchase supplements from trusted companies for safety.

If your gout pain is considerable, sudden, or intense — or if home remedies cease to work — contact your doctor immediately.

www.ingramcontent.com/pod-product-compliance
Lightning Source LLC
Chambersburg PA
CBHW070129260726
48658CB00001B/321